Think Out of belief

1, Volume 5

Dadhira Basumatary

Published by Dadhiram Basumatary, 2024.

Table of Contents

THINK OUT OF BELIEF

www.dadhirambasumatary.in

Chapter 1: Introduction

******

"Belief is a powerful thing, but it's even more powerful to question those beliefs."
  – Sadhguru

Get ready to hear an unbelievable narrative:

Throughout his journey, Mikel maintained an unshakeable belief, as unwavering as the towering peaks of the ancient Montana terrain that stood before him. The rugged landscape, with its jagged edges and majestic beauty, mirrored the firmness of his convictions. As the crisp mountain air filled his lungs, he felt a sense of clarity and purpose, like the pure scent of pine that permeated the surroundings.

Like the distant sound of a babbling brook, flowed through his veins and gave him the strength to navigate the challenges that lay ahead. Supported by his loving family, their unwavering presence was like a warm embrace that provided comfort and reassurance.

With unwavering optimism, he embraced each day as if it were a gift, believing in the inherent goodness of humanity. The vibrant colors of the wildflowers that dotted the valleys served as a constant reminder of the beauty that existed within people's hearts.

Yet, as life unfolded, it revealed a unique plan for Mikel, one filled with unforeseen twists and turns. The gusts of wind that swept through the vast open spaces whispered secrets of transformation, challenging his deeply held beliefs. It was here, amidst the grandeur of nature, that he found inspiration to embark on a journey of self-discovery and make profound changes within himself.

The journey began with what seemed to be a minor disruption: a slipped disc. Mikel's initial reaction was determined. Although the doctors deemed the surgery for his slipped disc a success, fate had more in store. Months later, Mikel experienced a suffocating chest pain that revealed a heart blockage, requiring urgent surgery. He approached this new challenge with the same faith that had guided him throughout his life, praying and hoping for the best. Yet, despite his fervent belief, the surgery failed, leaving him not only weakened but also devastated. Uncertainty, like a tiny bud, sprouted within him, growing into a vast expanse of disbelief.

The next setback came with the identification of cirrhosis, an ailment for which conventional treatment provided little expectation beyond managing the manifestations. Mikel's reality appeared to crumble. The person who once had faith in all aspects now questions them all. His confidence in contemporary healthcare completely broke. He felt lost, with each new therapy like a temporary cover on a hurt that ran deeper.

In a state of despair, Mikel turned to alternative treatments—herbal remedies, acupuncture, energy healing—but none provided the relief he sought. Each ineffective cure deepened his anguish, consuming him with the question, "Why me? "This question replaced his once-constant expressions of gratitude and hope."

Despite his growing skepticism, a glimmer of optimism persisted. The idea of his children maturing without him was unbearable. A glimmer of hope inspired him to explore beyond conventions and find new perspectives.

He learned about a mystic in India, a thinker outside of follower but seeker, whose wisdom blended ancient teachings with a modern understanding of the self. People reputed that this seeker, who was a thinker out of believer, practiced a form of holistic medicine that transcended mere physical healing. This appeared to be Mikel's last option, after losing faith in everything else.

Thus, in the last moments before his third surgery, he slipped away from his hospital bed. Without delay, Mikel embarked on a journey to

India, though his health made the trip arduous. Upon arrival, he sensed fatigue and a lack of direction. The individual who sees beyond belief but seeks, a symbol of calm presence, perceived beyond Mikel's physical suffering and acknowledged the deeper anguish within him—a man lost in turmoil.

The mindset of looking beyond being a believer but rather a seeker guided Mikel through a holistic approach that integrated body and spirit. Herbal remedies cleansed his body, while yoga and meditation nurtured his soul. Mikel learned the art of mindfulness from a seeker who taught him to embrace the present moment, letting go of past grievances and future anxieties.

Mikel went through a shift.

The persistent chest pain subsided, his breathing improved, and he experienced a newfound lightness. Over time, the liver cirrhosis, once deemed incurable, showed signs of reversal. Medication was no longer needed. Yet, the most profound transformation occurred within Mikel's mind and spirit. The mindset of a believer but seeker helped him understand that life's challenges are not mere obstacles, but growth opportunities. Mikel learned to embrace uncertainty, find strength in vulnerability, and rediscover a deeper faith—not just in external forces, but in his inner strength. As Mikel prepared to return home, he realized his journey had come full circle.

His global journey revealed the answers were always within. The act of introspection beyond belief, but as a seeker, had guided him to access his inner strength and wisdom. After returning to his family, Mikel was a different person. He renewed his spirit, and as a result, restored his health. He approached life with a new perspective, one that accepted both joy and sorrow with grace.

Mikel's story became a beacon of hope in his community, demonstrating the power of holistic healing, the resilience of the human spirit, and prizing deepening one's faith. Mikel's journey culminated in a profound self-discovery, surpassing mere physical

THINK OUT OF BELIEF

1. Cognitive Dimension

1. **What we believe:** This dimension represents the mental and intellectual aspects of belief. It focuses on how beliefs shape our understanding of reality, facts, and truth. It includes rationality, logic, and the ability to form judgments based on evidence.
2. **Example:** Believing that hard work leads to success is a cognitive belief based on reasoning or observation.

2. Emotional Dimension

1. **How we feel about our beliefs:** This dimension deals with the emotional attachment to our beliefs. It reflects the feelings that beliefs evoke, such as fear, hope, love, or anger. Often, beliefs are tied to deep emotions that can reinforce or challenge them.
2. Example: Belief in a higher power might evoke feelings of comfort, security, or awe.

3. Behavioral Dimension

1. **How beliefs influence our actions:** This dimension reflects how beliefs guide actions and behaviors. It addresses how our beliefs determine the decisions we make and how we live our lives.
2. Example: Someone who believes in environmental sustainability may adopt eco-friendly habits, like reducing plastic use or recycling.

4. Social Dimension

1. **How beliefs are shaped by and shape society:** This focuses

on how our beliefs are influenced by cultural, religious, social, and familial systems. It also explores how shared beliefs create communities and societal norms, shaping collective behavior.

2. Example: Cultural beliefs about gender roles can dictate what is considered "appropriate" behavior for men and women.

5. Spiritual Dimension

1. **Beliefs about meaning and existence:** This dimension pertains to beliefs concerning life's deeper meaning, purpose, and transcendence. It often deals with concepts of the divine, soul, morality, and existential questions.
2. Example: Beliefs in karma, reincarnation, or salvation reflect spiritual dimensions of belief.

6. Perceptual Dimension

1. How beliefs influence perception of reality: This dimension covers how our beliefs filter our perception of reality. Beliefs create biases and mental frameworks through which we interpret the world, often leading to selective attention or confirmation bias.
2. Example: Someone who believes the world is dangerous might perceive neutral events as threatening.

Other Possible Dimensions

1. **Philosophical Dimension:** Concerned with questions of "What is belief?" and "How can we know what we believe is true?"
2. **Epistemological Dimension:** Deals with how we come to form beliefs, especially in relation to knowledge, evidence, and truth.

THINK OUT OF BELIEF

Understanding belief across these dimensions reveals the complexity of how beliefs shape human experience, highlighting their multifaceted nature.

Why did I write this book? Do you eager to find out?

The act of writing a book is not merely to convey information, but to offer a transformative experience. So, why did I write this book? It is not just a collection of words—it is an invitation to join me on a journey. This book reflects my personal experiences and insights on the path to well-being. It delves into the physical, mental, and emotional challenges I've faced, the wisdom I've gained, and the methods I've discovered to elevate my quality of life.

Whether it's overcoming physical discomforts like foot pain or navigating the more subtle dimensions of the mind and emotions, the aim is to provide practical guidance for anyone think out of belief and seeking greater balance and vitality in their lives. Are you ready to walk this path with me?

It's about going beyond beliefs and understanding their interconnected dimensions. However, what I am writing focuses on one dimension—it's about uncovering a deeper sense of holistic well-being within yourself. It's about breaking free from the confines of belief and stepping into the realm of inner experience, where true transformation happens.

A transformation journey is more than weight loss or a new diet—it's about embracing a holistic way of living. I am Dadhiram Basumatary, editor, author, and publisher, and it is my privilege to guide you through this transformative process toward well-being.

Having personally experienced the challenges of weight—once standing at 213 pounds and finding my way to 163 pounds—I understand that these numbers reflect not just physical changes but a profound inner journey of growth and realization. You are not alone in this. Many, like you, have walked the path of think out of belief and seeking a healthier lifestyle, often feeling overwhelmed by countless diets, exercise routines, and temporary fixes.

But the journey we are thinking out of beliefs about to undertake together is not merely about losing weight; it's about discovering a more balanced and harmonious way of living. Take a moment to reflect on why you are here. Perhaps the weight you carry has become a burden, not just physically but emotionally. Maybe you've grown weary of seeing yourself in photos, or you're tired of struggling with unhealthy habits. I, too, faced these same challenges. It was my dissatisfaction with where I was that became the turning point, pushing me to think out of belief and think out of belief and seek lasting, holistic transformation rather than temporary solutions.

The conventional approach to weight loss often revolves around the simplistic idea of eating less and exercising more. While there may be some truth to this, it is a limited perspective. The journey we will take together goes beyond these surface-level approaches. This path is about understanding the interconnectedness of your mind, body, and emotions and creating a deeper, more sustainable approach to wellness. The holistic system we will explore is not just a set of rules; it is a way of integrating your entire being—your thoughts, emotions, and physical body—into a cohesive experience.

This journey is about more than just physical activity or dieting; it involves managing stress, adopting mindful eating habits, and understanding how your emotions shape your overall well-being. I invite you to imagine your future self—not just how you will look but how you will feel. Envision the confidence, the vitality, and the joy that comes with living a balanced life. Picture the inspiration you will provide to others, not just through your physical transformation but through the energy and presence you carry. This is not merely about appearance—it is about living fully and vibrantly.

The process itself is straightforward, but it requires dedication. The first step is to make a conscious decision to manage the stress that accompanies change. The second step involves replacing unhealthy habits with nourishing ones. Finally, the third step is to engage in physical activity that supports your holistic well-being, all while maintaining balance in your mind and emotions.

This book is your guide—a roadmap to holistic transformation. Together, we will explore the psychological, physiological, and emotional dimensions of wellness. Each chapter will build on the last, offering practical advice and tools to guide you toward a life of greater health and vitality. You will also receive valuable bonuses like a recipe guide and tips for managing emotional stress.

But remember, true transformation begins with a shift in mindset. Repeating the same actions and expecting different results will not bring lasting change. You must embrace new knowledge and apply it with intention. This holistic approach will guide you to sustainable success and a deeper sense of well-being. I welcome you to begin this journey with an open heart and mind. Read through these principles carefully. If they resonate with you, I look forward to walking this path together. If not, I still wish you to think out of belief well on your journey toward better health.

Welcome to the beginning of a new chapter in your life.

Summary: Take away tips:

Mikel's life was built on the solid foundation of faith, much like the towering mountains surrounding him. His unwavering beliefs gave him strength and shaped how he approached the world—with optimism and trust in life's goodness. However, life, in its unpredictable nature, challenged him at every step, forcing him to confront the limits of his belief system.

A series of health crises shook Mikel's world—first a slipped disc, then heart complications, and finally liver cirrhosis. Each time, Mikel faced these challenges with the same steadfast faith, but as surgery after surgery failed, doubt began to creep in. His rigid beliefs started to crack as his physical suffering deepened, leaving him disillusioned.

In desperation, Mikel turned to a mystic in India, embarking on a journey far from the traditional paths he had relied upon. It wasn't the mystic's knowledge of herbal remedies or alternative therapies that healed Mikel. It was the shift in perspective, the understanding that true healing lies not in external treatments but in inner transformation.

The mystic helped him see that life's hardships are not obstacles but opportunities for growth. Mikel learned to accept uncertainty, to live in the present moment, and to tap into a deeper source of faith—one that was not confined by rigid beliefs but expanded through awareness and inner strength.

Mikel's healing was not just physical. His journey led to a profound inner transformation. He returned to his family a renewed man, no longer clinging to fixed beliefs but open to the flow of life's experiences. Understanding that genuine faith transcends knowledge, he embraced the courage to question, think beyond belief, seek, and surpass it.

In view, Mikel's story illustrates that belief is not about certainty but about a willingness to evolve. It is not the external that limits us, but our own minds. When we let go of rigid beliefs and embrace the flow of life, we discover that all answers—and all healing—lie within us.

Chapter 2: Mind, Body, and Emotion.

******

Beliefs are just the stories we tell ourselves to justify our perceptions."
–Deepak Chopra

Why a Multidimensional Approach to Wellness?

Do you know what it means to embrace a multidimensional approach to wellness for long-term success? Let's revisit your first chapter. Today, we'll delve into the book and explore the concept of holistic living.

As you may recall from a previous overview of the course, chapter one focuses on establishing a sound foundation. We'll begin by defining what exactly "holistic" means and what it encompasses. So, without further ado, let's jump right in.

What is the typical approach to weight loss? According to traditional weight loss books, the key principles are eating less and exercising more. However, this outdated system's neglect of important aspects of well-being, such as mindfulness, calls for abandonment. A modern approach should consider all dimensions rather than solely focusing on one aspect, as traditional methods do. Maintaining a healthy lifestyle involves more than just one element.

Whether it's exercise, mindfulness, or diet, each plays an important role in achieving optimal health. Simply following a ketogenic or vegetarian diet, or engaging in vigorous exercise for hours each day, will not guarantee the desired results. Likewise, solely concentrating on the idea of having a lean body is not enough.

While some traditional weight loss books claim that one approach is sufficient, they overlook the fact that it takes a multifaceted approach to truly make a difference. It's not as simple as eating less and moving more. Traditional methods should no longer be considered relevant; they only cover one aspect and follow outdated guidelines.

It's time to expand our understanding of true holistic wellness and prioritize incorporating all components—nutrition, activity level, and mindset—into our routine for long-term success. Can you imagine what the book will provide you with? Recipes and valuable knowledge.

Simply eating is not enough; there are other important factors to consider. These recipes alone will not suffice. I will also provide you with an exercise program that will greatly improve your overall well-being, regardless of what you consume or how you manage your emotions.

Taking a one-dimensional approach, such as just meditating or changing your diet, may yield temporary results, but true success lies in addressing all aspects of your being—mind, body, and emotions. While it may seem appealing to focus solely on food or engage in extreme measures like surgery, these quick fixes only lead to disappointment in the long run. That's why taking a holistic approach is key. Holistic involves recognizing the bigger picture and understanding that one's identity encompasses more than just physical appearance and dietary choices. Embrace your mind, body, and emotions for sustainable wellness.

Figure 1

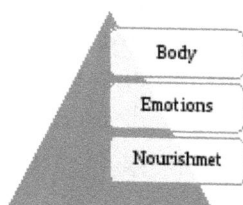

Multi-dimensional thinking is a complex concept that ties together the entirety of human existence. It highlights the interconnectedness of everything and everyone. In my opinion, this is the most crucial idea of the 21st century. Previously, the belief was that if you focused solely on your physical health, emotions, or diet, then you would be fine. However, that is only one aspect. You are not just a body, but rather a combination of body, emotions, and nourishment.

The holistic approach integrates all these elements to create a harmonious system that considers your body, emotions, and cognition.

The foundation of holistic living lies in this triangular approach, where all three components are harmonized for optimal well-being. In today's world, understanding this concept is essential for personal growth and fulfillment.

It's time to move away from one-dimensional thinking and recognize that we are more than just our physical bodies or emotional states. The holistic approach to living and thinking in ancient Vedic culture is centered around the concept of balance, which includes all aspects of oneself—body, mind, and emotions. 'Hat' is the name given to the balance triangle, where each side represents a crucial aspect of well-being. Equal sides are crucial for achieving triangle equilibrium.

Many solely focus on the biochemical component, which includes our food choices. However, neglecting the physiological and psychological aspects can leave this triangle distorted and incomplete. It is essential to pay attention to all sides to attain a true 'hat.' This is particularly relevant for gym enthusiasts who may not pay close attention to their habits and diet. It's common for them to think they can eat anything, but they often overlook the importance of knowing what ingredients go into their bodies and managing their emotions.

Unfortunately, I've witnessed some instructors at my gym who don't set a good example in this regard, even though they are supposed to guide us. They may have access to paid meals and feel that working out multiple times a day gives them the freedom to eat whatever they want, without considering the effects on their bodies and emotions. However, this is not the case. If you truly want a fit physique, you must be mindful of your food intake and how it fuels your body, as well as managing stress.

Another aspect to consider is whether you prioritize your spiritual or social well-being over physical health; I've seen this mindset among some individuals as well. The misconception about the Law of Attraction is a root cause. Many focus solely on visualizing and manifesting their desires without taking action or making necessary changes. However, this approach will not lead to the desired results.

So, how should you apply the triangle of holistic weight loss? All aspects must be addressed in a balanced triangle, not just one. Your physical body plays a crucial role, and therefore, movement is essential, as muscles can deteriorate without use. Let's not overlook the importance of managing your emotions, which can sabotage success and stem from various sources. We will discuss all three components of holistic health in depth later on.

It is crucial to consider your mind, emotions, and body when making choices about what to eat. This is the foundation we are building upon and a key concept to grasp in the 21st century. Pay attention to all three sides of the triangle—your body, mind, and emotions—as they are interrelated. This is the secret to achieving overall wellness.

Our solution can be summarized as follows: do not focus solely on one aspect while ignoring the others; this one-dimensional thinking will not lead to long-term success. Eating green leafy vegetables alone will not change your body shape, nor will simply going to the gym without taking care of your mental and emotional state. Mindfulness plays a significant role too—it's not just about physical exercise. Incorporating all three sides into your journey is essential for true holistic well-being.

The new approach is holistic, valuing both mind and body equally. Paying attention to all three aspects is key to achieving a healthy and successful change in body composition.

Losing weight may not necessarily result in a different body shape, so changing body composition should be the goal. This will lead to a more unified appearance and allow for fitting into smaller-sized clothes. Your triangle of health consists of your body, mindfulness, and motivation. In our next chapter, we will delve deeper into understanding your makeup and how your self-image affects your desired outcome.

As homework, grab a pen and paper and make three columns: Body, Mind, and Motivation. Write down changes needed for your well-being under each column. For example, under Body, you could write taking your bike to work or playing with your dog or children more often.

Category	Actions for Improvement
Body	Take the bike to work.
	Play with your dog or children more often.
	Incorporate more physical activities like walking or yoga.
Mind	Practice meditation or mindfulness daily.
	Take short breaks during work for mental relaxation.
	Engage in activities that stimulate your creativity or learning.
Emotions	Spend quality time with loved ones.
	Participate in activities that bring joy, such as hobbies or social events.
	Journal or express gratitude regularly.
Environment	Declutter your workspace and home for better focus.
	Surround yourself with positive and supportive people.

Table 1

This table provides a structure to focus on areas of life that contribute to overall well-being. I need to break out of my patterns and relax more to better handle stress and improve my nutrition. By reducing my intake of green coffee and cutting back on carbs and salt while incorporating more vegetables into my diet, I can make positive changes towards feeling better.

Take a moment to reflect on your own experiences and knowledge, noting any necessary adjustments or changes needed for a healthier lifestyle. I will give you two days to process this valuable chapter before you reconvene. It is crucial to truly understand and internalize this information for it to benefit you. Holistic living is the way of the future, so it's important to comprehend how it affects you and how you can implement it in your daily life by completing your assigned tasks. See you in two days.

Summary: Takeaway Tips:

Welcome to the first step of our journey, where we explore the depth of holistic living and its importance in achieving long-term success. Let's revisit the essence of our first chapter and delve deeper into what it means to embrace a multidimensional approach to wellness. Holistic living is not merely a trend, but a profound understanding that wellness encompasses all facets of our existence—mind, body, and emotions.

Traditional methods of weight loss often focus solely on reducing calories and increasing exercise. However, such a one-dimensional approach misses the essence of true well-being. Imagine if we only tended to one part of a garden while neglecting the rest. Neglecting the rest of the garden would compromise its overall health, even if the flowers still bloom. Similarly, focusing solely on diet or exercise without considering mental and emotional balance will not lead to sustainable wellness. A holistic approach integrates all dimensions of our being, recognizing that true health involves harmony across every aspect of life.

Our modern world demands a shift from outdated methodologies. Simply eating less or exercising more is not enough.

A complete understanding of wellness includes mindfulness, emotional stability, and physical health. The idea is to move beyond temporary fixes and embrace a lifestyle that addresses the whole person. Consider this: if your focus is solely on physical appearance, you may miss the crucial elements of mental clarity and emotional peace. These aspects are not separate but interwoven, influencing and supporting each other. Your well-being is like an equilateral triangle, where body, mind, and emotions must be equally nurtured for optimal health.

The concept of 'hat' in ancient Vedic culture represents this balance. Harmony of triangle sides creates equilibrium. Neglecting any side leads to distortion and imbalance. For instance, focusing solely on biochemical aspects like diet while ignoring emotional and psychological health will result in incomplete wellness. It is essential to address all aspects: what we consume, how we move, and how we manage our emotions. One-dimensional thinking, believing that eating right or exercising is sufficient, traps many people.

However, true transformation occurs when we approach wellness with a multifaceted mindset. This means integrating mindful practices, managing stress, and ensuring physical activity, rather than isolating each element. As you move forward, remember that holistic living is about seeing the bigger picture. It's about recognizing that you are a complex being whose health is influenced by a myriad of factors. Balancing your body, mind, and emotions is not just beneficial; it's essential for sustainable success and fulfillment. In our next chapter, we will dive deeper into how these elements interplay and how you can apply this understanding to your journey. Take a moment to ponder the interconnection of your well-being.

Consider making a list: Body, Mind, and Emotions. Under each category, jot down what changes or practices can bring balance and harmony into your life. Embrace this multidimensional approach and let it guide you toward a more profound and lasting transformation. Holistic living goes beyond concept, aligning with the essence of our existence. We will reconvene in two days, ready to explore in the second chapter how this understanding can further enhance your journey. Until then, may you see the interconnections within yourself and move toward a more balanced and fulfilling path?

Chapter 3: The Three Pillars of Success: Decision-Making, Action, and Perseverance in Holistic Weight Loss

******

"The mind that opens to a new idea never returns to its original size."
– Albert Einstein

Do you know about the Three Pillars of success: Decision-Making, action, and perseverance in Holistic Weight Loss?

Welcome back to Chapter Three. This is a crucial part of our course, and as mentioned earlier, it will provide you with three key factors for achieving success or failure. In our previous chapter, we discussed the ease of losing motivation and changing your physical appearance.

We also emphasized the importance of understanding and implementing these three pillars: decision-making under pressure, finding suitable substitutes for unhealthy habits, and incorporating physical movement into your routine. This book focuses on holistic living, encompassing both mind and body. It all starts with making a conscious decision, staying motivated, and being physically active. I hope this concept is clear now.

So, without further ado, let's dive into the first pillar of success: decision-making. A moment ago, the other two pillars include taking action and persevering toward your goals. What will bring you success? In this lesson, what does it mean to decide? It's determining how to achieve your desired outcome. You have a clear vision of what you want to accomplish—that's your decision. When you write it down, it becomes your goal—the thing you strive for.

Now, ask yourself: What appearance do I desire? What feelings do I want to experience? Is my concept unconventional? How do I envision my body, and what clothing size do I aspire to wear? To make a solid decision and turn it into a goal, start by pondering these questions and generating ideas about the result you desire. How would you like to feel about your body? As these questions arise, a mental image will take shape. You can write this picture once you form it, setting it as your goal.

However, to not only decide but also stick with it, it is essential to find your motivation. Why do you desire weight loss? What inspires you to change your body composition or appearance?

Identifying the benefits of this decision is crucial for success. How will losing weight and changing your body benefit you? You will feel even better than before. So why wait? Why delay this decision for months, years, or even five years? Procrastination will only delay progress. Therefore, it is vital to discover your reasons and motivations, as they will drive you toward achieving your goals.

It is important to pay attention to what you will need in the future. This key step involves visualizing and deciding on a course of action. My appearance has changed because of an unbalanced diet and sitting at work, and I'm tired of it. However, I refuse to accept this as my permanent state and am determined to make a change. To maintain motivation throughout the journey, I prioritize experiences over theory, recognizing the importance of firmly committing and acknowledging dissatisfaction with one's body.

Making an unbreakable decision is crucial to successfully transforming your body, regardless of any obstacles that may arise. What is necessary to transform your body? You must decide. Dissatisfied with my current appearance and actions, I aim to improve myself. After determining your goals, visualize how you want to feel. Think out of belief and seek guidance from your inner wisdom by asking yourself why you desire this change and what advantages it will bring. Consider what kind of clothing you want to wear and how you want to look at the beach. Once you make your decision, you hold on to the image created in your mind by these thoughts.

Figure 2

| 158 pound |
| 191 pound |
| 213 pound |

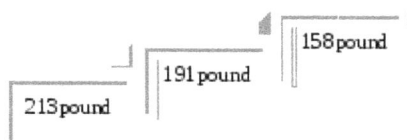

With this clear image, you can plan a goal statement such as "I am so happy and grateful now that I have a fit, healthy body." Will these actions lead to the envisioned future? Adding is key. Visualize and express gratitude for the image in your mind. For example, "I am delighted while wearing [an outfit] and feeling amazing" or "I am overjoyed now that I have a healthy weight of 158 pounds." Convert that visualization into a sentence, which is crucial, and jot it down on paper.

Consider setting a deadline by placing a question mark next to it. Should you establish guidelines? This decision is ultimately yours. It's worth considering if you have an upcoming event, such as a wedding or a terminal illness, in six months. Here, setting a deadline would be beneficial.

When facing a deadline, it's important to consider if there is truly something significant happening. If changing your belief is the goal, then focus on that. I didn't have anyone pushing me toward success, and it made me anxious thinking about living a wasted life. So, if a deadline only adds stress and anxiety to your plate, then perhaps it's best to reevaluate and make it your own goal instead. The result should feel content with yourself and living your best life possible. If giving yourself a deadline serves as motivation for an important goal, then by all means, go for it.

However, if there are no pressing deadlines or strict expectations in place, such as weight loss, then don't unnecessarily pressure yourself. Instead, follow your steps at your own pace, and you will achieve what you desire in due time. The initial task in this chapter is homework. Summarize it in a sentence and write it down.

Determine your goal and decide.

Imagine your goal and document it. I am filled with joy and gratitude now that you have a positive outlook on it. That is your long homework assignment. The second aspect of success is crucial, as it requires you to set your goal and make a firm decision about it. However, simply deciding is not enough if you do not take action towards achieving your goal.

Merely visualizing it in your mind will not bring it to readiness unless you put in the effort to turn it into reality. This means actively working towards it and taking the steps to make changes that align with your goal. So, what does taking action entail? It involves creating a plan by asking yourself: What steps do I need to take to reach my goal? What can I do right now to move towards my goal? Write these answers down on paper, and that becomes your plan of action. Remember, action starts from where you are right now, so begin anywhere and make progress towards your goal.

Summary: Take away tips

Welcome to the second chapter, where we unravel the essence of success through three fundamental pillars: Decision-Making, action, and perseverance. This chapter is pivotal in your journey, as these principles are not just theoretical concepts but practical steps toward holistic weight loss. Let's begin with decision-making. Deciding is not merely choosing from options but setting a clear intent for your life.

It is an acknowledgment of your current state and a commitment to change. Ask yourself: What is the image of yourself that you desire? What feelings do you want to experience in your body? This image you create in your mind becomes your goal. Write it down, see it, and own it. A decision's strength depends on the resolve behind it.

Your deepest motivation must be back in it. Why do you believe in and pursue this change? What will it bring into your life? This inner drive is what will propel you forward. Moving to the next pillar, action. It is one thing to see, but quite another to manifest it. Action is the bridge between your decision and the reality you wish to create. It involves not just planning but executing those plans with dedication.

What steps will you take today to move closer to your goal?

Document these steps and take action from where you stand. Every small action is a step toward transforming your vision into reality. Last, there's perseverance. This is the force that keeps you moving forward despite obstacles. It's about maintaining your course even when the journey seems challenging. Understand that success is not instantaneous but a culmination of consistent effort.

Even when motivation wanes, perseverance ensures that your actions continue, and your goals remain within reach. In this journey, visualize your goal, act on it with determination, and persevere through the highs and lows. Your mind and body are not separate entities, but a unified force. When you align your thoughts, actions, and persistence, you pave the way for true transformation. So, let's embark on this journey in Chapter 4 with rational decisions, deliberate actions, and unwavering perseverance. These four pillars illuminated your path to success, guiding you toward holistic and fulfilling change.

Chapter 4: Unlocking the Power of Your Mind for Weight Loss Success

****

"To believe something because it is fashionable is the height of stupidity."
    –Voltaire

How to Unlock the Power of Your Mind for Successful Weight Loss.

Welcome to this profound chapter 3 of exploration. We are not merely talking about the mechanics of vehicles or how they function externally. Here, we are delving deeper into the psychological vehicle—this body-mind complex.

Today, we shall investigate the intricate dynamics of self-image, the workings of the conscious and subconscious mind, and how they steer our life's journey. This is not a small inquiry because the way your mind functions determines the trajectory of your life—whether it moves forward effortlessly or stumbles over obstacles.

Let me first share a minor story from my life. You may look at me now and think, "Ah, this man seems fine, at peace, even in this body." But life was not always this way for me. I remember a time long ago—1989, to be exact—when I had just taken up a new job. Back then, I was slim and energetic, weighing only 163 pounds. But over time, as life happens, with duties pulling in different directions, my weight crept up. Eight years later, by 1997, I carried 213 pounds on this frame. I had never experienced such a change in my body before, and I found it rather embarrassing.

But you see, I did not sit around making excuses or blaming the universe. I recognized the need for change, both inside and outside. The moment you decide that something must change, a new possibility arises. Both the body and mind serve as instruments, not obstacles. Your mind, when used well, becomes your greatest asset. But first, you must understand how it operates.

Let us begin with the mind itself. Many people think their brain and their mind are the same. Yet, the brain is nothing more than a complex, physical organ made of meat. The mind, however, is much more subtle. It controls your brain like an orchestra conductor.

Two main aspects of the mind are conscious and subconscious. The conscious mind is what you use for planning, reasoning, and navigating daily life. But beneath this surface is the vast ocean of your subconscious mind. This is where your habits, deepest values, and lifelong memories live. It is this subconscious mind that often runs the show without you even realizing it.

Your body, too, is not just flesh and bone. The mind and body have a strong connection. The interplay influences your very heartbeat, the way your immune system responds, and the way you carry yourself — between your conscious and subconscious mind. You may think it is willpower or discipline alone that changes your body, but in truth, your body remembers. It remembers everything—every habit, every meal, and every choice. And so, real transformation happens when both the conscious and subconscious minds align toward a goal.

In ancient traditions, specifically Vedic sciences, the mind is known to possess four dimensions. These are not merely psychological concepts; they represent different aspects of your being. First, there is "buddhi," or intellect. Then, "ahankara," or identity. Next comes "manas," which we can call memory. Finally, there is "Chitta," pure intelligence, untouched by memory or identity. Each dimension impacts who you are and your life experience.

The problem in today's world is that we have become overly reliant on intellect alone. Our belief is that resolving matters mentally will bring about a favorable outcome. Life surpasses this simplicity. Your identity—what you associate yourself with—often governs your intellect. If you identify yourself in a limited way, whether by nationality, religion or even body image, your intellect will work to protect that identity, often at the expense of your well-being.

Memory, or manas, is even more profound. Your entire body carries the memory of not just this lifetime, but perhaps many lifetimes before. It stores the memory of every experience and action, shaping how you respond to the world.

Beyond all this is Chitta—pure, unblemished intelligence. This is where the real magic lies. When you tap into this dimension, you move beyond intellect and memory into a space of creation. Here, real transformation becomes possible—not just of your body, but of your entire experience of life.

How can we bring about this change? First, it begins with a change in perception. If you want to change your body, you must first change the way you see yourself. When you look in the mirror, what is it that you see?

If you see yourself as overweight, unfit, or unattractive, this perception becomes a reality in your mind. But what if, instead, you see yourself as healthy, vibrant, and full of energy? Visualize your desired body daily, with ease and happiness.

You see, your mind holds tremendous power. If you consistently hold a new image in your mind's eye—an image of the body you wish to create—slowly but surely, your subconscious will align with this vision. It will bring about the changes necessary to manifest this reality. It may take time—21 days, perhaps, or more—but if you stick with it, you will see the transformation unfold. This is not merely about weight loss or physical appearance. Harmonize your mind and body with your desired life.

Set aside a few minutes each day to calmly sit, close your eyes, and visualize your new self. Smile, feel the joy of this vision, and let it seep into your subconscious. Speak kindly to yourself, for your words carry power. Affirm your well-being with simple statements like, "I love my body," "I am healthy," or "I am transforming." These are not just empty words.

Repeated often enough, these thoughts reshape your subconscious, rewiring it towards health and vitality. You must understand—your body is just the surface. What truly matters is how you hold your mind. How can your body reflect anything but negativity, doubt, and self-criticism if you fill your mind with them?

If positivity, love, and purpose reside in your mind, the body will naturally align. Please make a daily effort to connect with this vision. Make it a habit and a joyful part of your routine: just five minutes in front of the mirror, smiling at yourself and visualizing your best self. This is not just vanity; it is a sacred practice of self-creation.

As you go about your day, carry these affirmations with you. Whenever you feel doubt creeping in, replace it with a positive thought. Over time, this will become second nature, and you will see your body—your entire life—transform in ways you never imagined. So, let us begin this journey together. You have everything you need within you. Your mind, your body, your very energy—they are all tools, waiting for you to take charge. Visualize, affirm, and above all, be kind to yourself. When you align your mind with your deepest intentions, there are no limits to what you can achieve.

In our previous chapter 2, we touched upon something fundamental—the inner workings of the conscious and subconscious mind. Understanding this is pivotal for weight loss or any life goal. You see, what you consciously think and believe becomes the nourishment for your subconscious mind.

It is like feeding seeds to fertile soil; the quality of those seeds will determine what grows within you. If we sow thoughts of limitation and fear, our subconscious mind will work tirelessly to manifest them. But if we plant seeds of clarity, confidence, and self-worth, our subconscious will create a life of balance and well-being.

This chapter explores the hidden depths of self-sabotage. Now, what do I mean by self-sabotage? It is the condition where, despite your best intentions and efforts, some unseen force within you seems to hold you back. It's almost as if you are pressing the accelerator while also keeping your foot on the brake. You may feel that you're working diligently toward a goal, but deep within, something is quietly obstructing your progress.

THINK OUT OF BELIEF

Dear one, the mind operates at two levels: conscious and subconscious. The conscious mind is like the captain of a ship, deciding and giving commands. But the subconscious mind is the engine room, tirelessly following the captain's orders without ever questioning them.

If the captain is not clear or sends mixed signals, the engine room may follow misguided instructions, steering the ship into uncharted and even dangerous waters. Therefore, awareness of your inner dialogue is essential.

If you focus your conscious mind on achieving a goal, but your subconscious mind harbors old patterns of doubt, fear, or trauma beneath the surface, the two will be at odds. The result? You'll feel stuck, life not flowing as it should. This is the essence of self-sabotage. Now, let us explore why this happens. Lack of effort or discipline isn't always the cause. Sometimes, it stems from deeper psychological reasons—perhaps unprocessed traumas or unresolved emotions.

People struggling with weight or self-image may feel unsafe due to negative past experiences. In response, the body adopts a kind of protective mechanism, storing weight to shield itself from unwanted attention. In such cases, the subconscious mind is not sabotaging you maliciously; it is trying to protect you based on experiences, even though those experiences are no longer relevant.

For example, some people avoid exercise not because they lack motivation but because they have associated physical activity with trauma or fear. I have witnessed this myself.

Many years ago, during a public event, I saw a beloved actor, Puneeth Rajkumar, collapse and pass away right in front of digital eyes. Witnessing that moment shocked me, keeping me away from gyms for nearly a decade. Every time I saw gym equipment, I would recall that traumatic experience. The body remembers, and it responds accordingly.

These psychological and physiological barriers can be very real, but they are not insurmountable. This brings us to the practical aspect of overcoming self-sabotage. First, you must realize how you are sabotaging yourself.

To gauge this, simply think about your goal, whether it's weight loss, fitness, or anything else. Ask yourself, on a scale of 0 to 10, how does this goal make you feel? If it provokes a feeling of intense stress (let's say 6 or above), you are likely holding onto self-sabotaging patterns.

These patterns could manifest as procrastination, fear of failure, or even success aversion. If the stress level is lower than 6, it may just be normal stress, the kind that comes with any effort to bring about change. Yet, if it surpasses that, further work is required.

So, how do we address this? One simple yet profound technique is to focus on releasing this internal stress. Visualization is a powerful tool. Picture in your mind the body or life you desire—something lean, healthy, and vibrant.

Now, while holding this image, lightly tap the bone under your eyes and focus on your breath. This gentle tapping helps release tension and blockages in your body. As you breathe deeply and visualize your goal, you will probably feel a subtle but noticeable shift—a sense of lightness, as though something is being released.

Ask yourself again: how does the goal feel now? Has the stress reduced? Any decrease in stress levels, even from 10 to 6 or 4, signifies progress. You are breaking through the layers of self-sabotage that have held you back. With regular practice, these self-sabotaging patterns will slowly dissolve, and your mind and body will work in harmony.

However, let us not overlook the broader context of stress in life.

However, let us not overlook the broader context of stress in life. Stress comes in many forms—financial struggles, relationship difficulties, past traumas, and daily pressures. When stress becomes chronic, it not only affects your mental health but also takes a toll on your physical body.

THINK OUT OF BELIEF

High blood pressure, headaches, insomnia, weight fluctuations, and digestive problems are just a few of the physical manifestations of unresolved stress. Emotionally, stress can lead to depression, anxiety, and a feeling of helplessness. Therefore, adopting practices to reduce stress is crucial for both the mind and body.

Techniques like the ones we discussed—tapping, deep breathing, and visualization—are highly effective. They allow you to release tension from your body, reprogram your subconscious mind, and align it with your conscious goals. In summary, dear one, your mind consists of two parts: the conscious mind, where you set goals and intentions, and the subconscious mind, which quietly operates in the background, carrying out the instructions it receives.

Hidden beliefs or unprocessed emotions buried in the subconscious can act as roadblocks, sabotaging even your best efforts. However, by realizing these patterns and practicing techniques to release them, you can overcome these barriers and move toward success with greater ease.

Remember, stress is an inevitable part of life, but how we handle it makes all the difference. Engage in practices that bring balance to your mind, body, and emotions. As you implement these methods, you will notice a significant shift in your energy and clarity. Physical homework not necessary for this chapter. Put our discussions into practice for transformative change. I look forward to seeing how you progress as you clear these mental and emotional roadblocks and move toward a life of balance, well-being, and success.

Summary: Takeaway Tips:

The mind is a magnificent instrument. It holds within it both the conscious and the subconscious; they saw and the unseen, the known and the unknown. Like an iceberg, the conscious mind is just a tip. But below this surface lies the vastness of the subconscious, an ocean of memories, habits, and beliefs that silently shape our lives.

When we speak of transformation, especially in matters of weight loss or health, it is not just about physical action. It is about reshaping the very foundation of how we perceive ourselves. Your self-image is more than just a mirror reflection.

This self-image often comes from old memories, experiences, and deeply held beliefs that guide your behavior without you even knowing. If you wish to change—if you truly wish to transform—you must first look within.

The subconscious mind is like fertile soil; whatever you plant there will grow. If you plant the seeds of doubt, fear, and failure, they will manifest in your life. But if you plant the seeds of self-love, strength, and clarity, these too will blossom into reality.

Your body is not separate from your mind. It responds to every thought, every emotion, every belief. Aligning the body and mind starts with aligning the conscious and subconscious. It's not a battle, it's a dance. Your self-perception extends beyond the mirror. The conscious mind must steer the subconscious with clarity and purpose, like a ship's captain. In doing so, the ship—the body—follows naturally. Do not underestimate the power of visualization.

When you see yourself as strong, healthy, and vibrant, this image takes root in the subconscious. Slowly, the body will follow. Yet, it is not solely about the act of seeing; Whatever you believe about yourself is what will unfold in your life. Each day, find time to sit, breathe, and visualize your desired self. Allow this image to fill not just your mind, but your entire being.

THINK OUT OF BELIEF

In this process, you find that the transformation you believe in is not external. Namaskar, and may you find the strength to guide your ship with wisdom and grace? In Chapter 5, you may understand who you are in harmony with; as you do, you become capable of living fully, and health follows as a natural consequence

Chapter 5: Consciously Shaping Habits.

******

"The greatest enemy of knowledge is not ignorance; it is the illusion of knowledge."
 – *Stephen Hawking*

What Role Does the Conscious Mind Play in Shaping Habits?

Do you know the intricate dance of life? What is the role of the mind? In Chapter 4, we discussed the psychological aspects of weight loss and delved into the conscious and subconscious mind's memories. We explored the impact of self-image on our actions and thoughts. Our subconscious operates based on what our conscious mind feeds it, so it's crucial to monitor what we allow into our thoughts.

In this important chapter, we'll focus on identifying and overcoming self-sabotaging thought patterns. This is a topic I'm personally passionate about, and I hope you'll find it intriguing as well. Remember, your mind has two parts: the conscious and the subconscious. The conscious mind commands, the subconscious obeys unquestioningly. So be careful of what you feed your mind, because it will determine how your subconscious responds.

As the captain of your ship, you have control over your life and mind, while the subconscious simply follows your lead without questioning it. That's why paying attention to your self-talk and self-image is vital in achieving your goals.

Now let's shift our focus to Chapter 3, where we dive into the topic of self-sabotage. Despite your best efforts, you may find yourself not seeing the desired results. This can be confusing and frustrating; you have a simple plan and are working toward your goals, but something seems to hold you back.

It may not be entirely your fault. Earlier in Chapter 4, there are subconscious mind factors at play that can hinder even our most determined efforts. These factors operate below our conscious experiences of memories, causing us to sabotage ourselves without even realizing it.

Repeated failures and unexplained obstacles can manifest. You may be diligently following all the steps I've outlined so far, taking no shortcuts, yet still wonder why success eludes you. The answer lies in these hidden inner workings of your mind—one part of you is striving for progress while another is unknowingly hindering you. It's a delicate balance between your conscious desires and subconscious patterns that can make or break your journey toward your goal.

Your current results may not be meeting your expectations. If you have experienced past traumas, such as sexual assault or shame, it's difficult to believe that looking attractive will not lead to similar situations happening again. Here, you may choose to maintain a larger body size to avoid unwanted attention and keep others at a distance.

This can also affect your relationships, causing you to feel pressure to provide physical intimacy as a way of compensating for experiences. If you struggle with self-love, food may become a source of comfort instead. Ultimately, these psychological factors may prevent you from wanting to lose weight. There are a variety of reasons someone may not want to engage in exercise, including physiological problems.

Possible causes include injury, post-workout trauma, and exercise-related psychological issues. I have experienced this firsthand. A few years ago, while at the gym, everyone in India witnessed the collapse of a famous South Indian film actor, who died right in front of everyone. Witnessing his life fade and his face distort traumatized me, keeping me away from the gym for ten years. Even now, the sight of an ambulance or specific gym equipment can induce anxiety and avoidance.

Other people also struggle with psychological barriers such as low self-esteem or short- and long-term illnesses that interfere with their ability to exercise regularly. There may also be physiological issues, such as muscle or tendon injuries, that prevent physical activity, along with biochemical imbalances in the body.

Food-related factors can play a role, such as allergic reactions or difficulties with binge eating. These challenges span across the three prongs of the mind-body connection: psychological, physiological, and biochemical problems that can affect our relationship with exercise and overall well-being.

Subcultures can be a factor in self-sabotage in urban areas. To determine if you are actively sabotaging yourself, simply consider your current goal and ask yourself how it makes you feel on a scale of 0 to 10. Don't overthink it; just trust your initial response. If your goal provokes a high level of stress (6 or above), you have active self-sabotaging thoughts running through your mind.

This might cause panic or overwhelm. However, if your stress level is lower than 6, you may simply experience normal stress related to the unknowns and changes involved in pursuing your goal. But if it is 6 or above, you likely have active self-sabotaging thoughts holding you back from achieving your goal.

So, what can be done? If you rate your stress as 6 or higher, you likely have psychological barriers caused by active self-sabotaging thoughts in your mind. Here, consider taking the following steps:

Picture in your mind the body you desire—a nice, lean, toned physique. Sit cross-legged in a yoga position, close your eyes, and begin tapping in a mudra position, not too tight or too loose. Focus on your breathing while envisioning your improved image. Continue tapping until you feel a release throughout your body. Keep your eyes closed and maintain the image in your mind. You may experience a feeling of relief, as if someone has lifted a weight off you.

Breathe out and open your eyes. Now, go back to that image and ask yourself how it makes you feel. Is there any stress? Our goal is to reduce image stress, even if it drops to a 4 from a 10, that's progress! Don't worry about any remaining stress, as we can work on it later. The important thing is that it has lessened, and by consistently doing this exercise, it will continue to decrease until self-sabotaging thoughts are no longer present.

Now, let's talk about stress—it is simply the result of having to adapt or change our lives. Every time we decide or take action towards change, we experience some level of stress. There is a potential for positivity. This topic involves change and might lead to stress. Various factors, such as financial issues, can cause this type of stress, relationship struggles, past trauma, or other personal circumstances.

These sources of stress are harmful to our overall well-being, as they affect us physically and emotionally. Some common physical effects include high blood pressure, infections, diabetes, headaches, muscle tension, insomnia, weight gain or loss, constipation, dizziness, and sexual problems. Emotional stress can cause depression and low self-esteem or cause us to feel overwhelmed or in denial. It may also lead to a lack of productivity and make us more prone to accidents.

You might remember moments when stress caused you to drop things or have minor accidents because of being distracted. In severe cases, people may turn to workaholism or substance abuse to cope with stress, which can eventually lead to burnout. Allowing stress to take over our lives can have negative effects on our physical appearance as well. To combat this problem, it is important to decrease stress levels. In the previous section, I showed an effective technique known as Emotional Stress Relieving (ESR). Let's now inspect.

How can you feel better?

How can you feel better? Numerous approaches exist, similar to those depicted in media. It's hard to believe, but these seemingly insignificant points play a major role in relieving stress unconsciously. Our bodies have a clever design that targets these points and helps us feel better.

You can also try this technique at work, especially when you're sitting at your desk all day. Place two fingers lightly on the designated points and take deep breaths. As you breathe, you'll notice a sense of calmness and relaxation. Evaluate stress level, post recovery, on a scale of 0 to 10. If it's too high (above 6), try using the tapping technique to further reduce stress and self-sabotage patterns.

In summary, our memory has both conscious and subconscious parts. The conscious part is where we plan and set goals, while the subconscious works behind the scenes without our controlled awareness. Hidden beliefs can interfere with our goals even when we try to achieve them. Keep practicing this method whenever you feel stressed and use it as a tool for personal growth. As an individual, it is crucial to take care and be mindful of your emotional stress levels in various situations.

One effective technique to reduce stress and eliminate any sabotage caused by negative thoughts is tapping. Stress is inevitable in our daily lives, but that does not mean we should let it consume us. If not addressed, it can harm our physical and mental well-being. However, avoiding society's demands is not the solution. Engaging in techniques like holding the fort can further decrease stress in all aspects of life where dissatisfaction arises.

This chapter contains valuable information, so it may be helpful to revisit it at a later time. These techniques will greatly impact the outcome, and no written homework is required.

By using tapping, you can gain a better understanding of your thoughts and break through any psychological barriers preventing you from achieving your goals. The good news is that with these techniques, you can relieve stress and eliminate any roadblocks in your path toward success. I look forward to seeing your progress this time around!

Summary: Take away tips

Ah, in the intricate dance of life, the mind holds sway over the body in ways most of us cannot grasp. You see, when we speak of weight loss or transformation, it is not simply the body that we must address. It is just a vessel, the body. The true essence of action lies within the mind, with its multiple layers. The conscious mind, as a ship's captain, chooses the destination.

But the subconscious steers the ship through the ocean of life with unwavering dedication, regardless of the direction it receives. Now, if we have programmed the subconscious with fears, past wounds, or limiting beliefs, it may unknowingly sabotage even our most earnest efforts.

The conscious mind, like a captain setting sail toward the horizon, can strive for greatness while the subconscious mind keeps us tethered to old patterns. This is the root of self-sabotage. The scars of past traumas, the fears of being seen or judged, and the resistance to change — all these things lodge themselves in the depths of the subconscious, subtly guiding our choices, our habits, and our very desires.

To comprehend the mind's nature and acknowledge its sustenance is crucial. Every thought, every word - a seed. What we feed the subconscious becomes our reality. When you feed your thoughts with doubt, fear, or unworthiness, your subconscious will diligently create a life that mirrors that belief.

However, if we can shift these patterns and rewrite the narrative that plays within, then true transformation is possible. So, we do not merely wage a battle of diet and exercise. First, cleanse and align the mind with our desired vision. Then, dissolve self-sabotage barriers.

To do this, one must sit, still as a mountain, and breathe life into a new image of themselves. Imagine a lighter body, heart, and mind -

not just in theory, but in reality. To seek change externally, we must first cultivate it internally.

Once you become the conscious master of your inner ship, guiding the subconscious with clarity and purpose, you will no longer find yourself bound by the old ways. You will flow toward your goal effortlessly. So, be mindful of your thoughts, for they are the architects of your reality.

Chapter 6: The Journey to a Healthier You: Understanding Biochemical Components of Weight Loss.

******

Your desires lie beyond fear's grasp, claims George.

them consistently because simply knowing about them won't bring any change. Now, let's address what could be hindering your progress. The first step is making a firm decision and handling the accompanying stress. In the previous chapter, this is crucial. Moving on to the second step—learning how to replace unhealthy nutrition habits with healthier ones—is what Chapter 5 focuses on.

Why is experience important?

Why does experience matter? Achieving fitness and well-being goes beyond physical effort—it requires aligning body, mind, and energy. In 1987, life placed me in the corporate world when I joined an oil company that later merged with one of India's Navaratna enterprises. The external success and prestige of the job came with its own set of challenges, including the biases and discrimination I faced, even among educated circles. But life has its way of teaching us through obstacles, and I persisted.

However, a pivotal moment came when my frustration with modern medicine peaked. It was during the pregnancy of my second child. Our company doctor prescribed an X-ray test just days before my wife's delivery to confirm if she was carrying twins. My young daughter, Jirina, was struggling with a severe case of tonsillitis, and the doctors recommended surgery to remove the infected portion of her throat. It felt like we were becoming prisoners of modern medicine.

Meanwhile, my body had been changing in ways that concerned me. I had grown from 163 pounds to 213 pounds—perhaps because our diet resembled the American USDA food pyramid, a pattern that emphasizes carbohydrates over fats and proteins. This, along with an unfortunate scooter accident that led to a lumbar infection, stirred something deeper within me. I realized that modern medicine, while effective in certain scenarios, was not providing the holistic solution I sought. It seemed like my reliance on it was pulling me further away from true well-being.

Amidst the crisis, I averted my gaze. I turned to alternative medicine, specifically homeopathy. I found a homeopath, Subash Dev, and began exploring this ancient method of healing for both me and my family. This shift allowed me to transcend conventional medicine's limitations and take charge of my health.

THINK OUT OF BELIEF

This journey to health goes beyond pills and food. It's about knowing your body and nature.

The modern diet, full of excess carbohydrates, is just one example of how disconnected we have become from the natural ways of sustaining life. Through my trials with health, I discovered the immense benefits of taking a holistic approach—where body, mind, and spirit work in unison.

Please understand that I share this without any heroic intentions. I never rose to fame or fortune through the corporate ladder, and there is nothing legendary in the external sense. But looking back,

I realize that the real accomplishment lay in discovering something unfamiliar too many—the capacity to help others by transforming my life first. I found my true mission: to serve, to uplift, and to share these insights with others. The insights I share in this book are born of these experiences. I hope they help you unlock your potential, just as they helped me find mine.

We all face challenges, setbacks, and moments of despair, but the quality of our habit's shapes life's quality. If we continue with the same habits, we will achieve the same outcomes. But if we cultivate better habits, the possibilities are limitless. I know many people might claim to achieve success overnight.

I have met none of them, and I am certainly not one of them. There was no single defining moment when everything changed for me. My journey was not from one diet fad to the next; it wasn't about hopping from Paleo to Keto. The evolution was gradual, trying everything, learning from experiences, and breaking through step by step.

Through persistence, I found my way back to a healthier weight—167 pounds—and a balanced blood pressure of 120/80 of mm Hg. It was not a miracle, but a series of small, consistent steps. Starting small was my only option. Eventually, these small steps culminated in something much larger—a holistic lifestyle aligned with the body's natural rhythms and the mind's clarity.

Now, with this book and my upcoming coaching business (which I plan to launch in December 2024), I wish to share these lessons with you. There is no shortcut to real success, but there is a way—a path that requires you to start small, stay consistent, and remain mindful of your body's needs. Health and well-being are not destinations; they are the ongoing result of conscious living.

Do you yearn to discover the vivid details of my AHA moment?

Are you eager to know my AHA moment? Let me share: the ancient concept of karma—the understanding that what goes around comes around—can profoundly influence the course of our lives. One such moment of transformation occurred for me in October 2019 when I received selection for a 15-day training program in Modern Sericulture Processing Technology at Zhejiang Sci-Tech University in Hangzhou, China. It went beyond being a professional experience.

Along with my colleague, I embarked on our trip from Guwahati airport, traveling through Kolkata to Nanjing, and then to Hangzhou. Upon our arrival at the beautiful Zhejiang Hotel, we immersed ourselves in the local environment and food culture. It was during this time that I became deeply curious about the differences between Indian and Chinese food, especially regarding health and well-being.

One thing that struck me during my stay in China was the rarity of seeing obese people. Most people were slim and fit, and I soon realized that their food habits were a significant factor. I followed their diet strictly for the duration of my stay and committed to continue these habits when I returned.

However, when I returned in November 2019, the outbreak of the coronavirus pandemic hit the world. We had to confine ourselves at home and limit our social interactions because of the imposed lockdowns. This period presented a challenge to maintaining the disciplined eating habits I had adopted in China.

Our diets are heavily reliant on carbohydrates—18 ounces to 21 ounce per meal—with minimal protein and fat and little to no fruits and nuts. I realized that to transform my health; I needed to reduce my carbohydrate intake drastically. Back in 2019, I weighed 213 pounds and struggled with severe knee pain, high blood pressure, back pain, and sleep disturbances. These issues were exacerbated by feelings of lethargy, a lack of confidence, and the inability to engage in physical activities, like jogging or morning walks.

I had tried various methods—joining jogging clubs, yoga sessions, gyms, and even swimming—but nothing seemed to work. Each attempt at a new routine led to a return to old habits and increased weight. Doctors advised surgery for my back pain, but I was determined to avoid that route. Instead, I sought relief through Ayurvedic massage, which helped to some extent, but I knew there was something deeper that needed to be addressed.

Our diet predominantly comprises carbohydrates, with white rice being a staple. I was consuming nearly 28 ounces of rice every day, supplemented by a small amount of protein and fat. They ingrained in me that without carbs, survival would be difficult.

However, I questioned this mindset, especially as I noticed the rise of chronic diseases like diabetes, cancer, and obesity in our society. During my time at Zhejiang University, someone introduced me to a radically different diet.

The university canteen served balanced meals, consisting of about 4 ounces of carbs, 2 ounces of protein (both plant-based and animal-based), 2 ounces of salad, 2 ounces of mixed vegetables, and one whole fruit. I strictly followed this diet for the 21 days I was in China and felt significantly lighter and healthier. I resolved to continue this practice upon returning to India, despite the challenges of accessing the same food.

In this journey, I developed what I call the "3-in-1 Method of Holistic Fitness," focusing on three key areas: the mind (mental and emotional well-being), the body (physical health), and the spirit (attitude). This holistic approach was essential to my transformation.

Controlling my mind was the initial step. Back in 2015, when I weighed 213 pounds, I felt hungry, lethargic, and lacked confidence. My diet was carb-heavy, with little protein, fat, fruits, or vegetables.

However, after my experience in China, I embraced a balanced diet—one-third of carbohydrates, one-third protein, and one-third vegetables, fruits, and fats. I stuck to a new eating regimen for 21 days and promptly noticed increased energy and a lighter feeling.

I continued this regimen for nine months after returning home, and by the end of the journey, I had shed 50 pounds, going from 213 pounds to 163 pounds. The transformation succeeded in mind, body, and energy.

Ancient wisdom regarding the connection between the body, mind, and energy goes beyond modern science, reaching into the essence of life itself. It speaks of the body and mind as intertwined expressions of the same life energy. The connection between body and mind is not new. Ancient wisdom traditions have explored this truth. Modern quantum physics provides an interesting lens to understand it.

Quantum theory suggests that all matter comprises minuscule particles called quanta, which remain in a state of potential until someone observes or measures them. This means the simple act of observation can alter the behavior of matter.

The body-mind relationship is strengthened by the mutual influence of the mind's energy on the body, and vice versa. The mind's energy is a potent force, as wisdom emphasizes.

What you think and how you focus your mental energy can shape not only your emotions but also your physical well-being. Studies have shown that positive thinking and mental visualization can create actual changes in the body, reducing pain, lowering blood pressure, and strengthening the immune system.

This supports the idea that the mind's energy can impact the body at a quantum level. Traditional practices such as acupuncture, Reiki, and qigong have worked with this understanding of energy for centuries. Methods rely on energy flow through body, imbalances or blockages cause illness.

By realigning this energy, one can restore health and vitality. Healing involves balancing life energies that govern the body and mind, as per this wisdom. The body surpasses being a mere machine, and the mind goes beyond mere thoughts. They both express the same life energy.

Understanding this connection opens up a new way of approaching health—one that recognizes the profound influence on our consciousness has on our physical state. Healing, from this perspective, is about aligning body, mind, and energy in harmony.

Summary: Take away tips

Summary: As you leave, here are some important take away tips to remember.

In the intricate dance of life, the body functions not as a machine but as a beautiful balance of energies. People should understand that weight loss is not merely about cutting calories or punishing the body into shape.

Food is not just sustenance; it is memory, both physical and emotional. Every bite you take carries the impressions of your past, influences your present, and shapes your future. The process of losing weight is not a battle to be fought; it is a harmony to be created within yourself.

You see, it's not about restrictions; it's about relationships—your relationship with food, your body, and your mind. As you delve into the depths of your biochemical makeup, you see that the power lies within you to bring balance.

Replacing old habits with nourishing ones is not an act of deprivation but of awakening—a conscious choice to fuel your body with what it truly needs to thrive.

As you begin your transformative journey, let go of belief and the need to control your body.

Align with life's flow through understanding and let go of the unnecessary. What you eat, how you move, and the decisions you make - these are the sacred dance of well-being.

May this journey not only change your body but also awaken a deeper connection to the vast intelligence that sustains you.

This is not a fight against yourself; it is a return to your true nature, and you will gain a deeper understanding of dietary choices in Chapter 7.

Chapter 7: Exploring Dietary Styles and Choices.

****

"Progress is impossible without change, and those who cannot change their minds cannot change anything." – George Bernard Shaw.

How can one go about exploring various dietary styles and choices?

Welcome to Chapter 7, where we will discuss dietary styles and types. Let's begin by delving into the biochemical components of nutrition and food. As we have explored in previous chapters, three main diets eliminate specific components, such as gluten, dairy, and carbohydrates.

These diets can be personal choices rather than medical necessities. Ultimately, the best motivation for maintaining a healthy diet is to consume whole, unprocessed foods that you prepare yourself.

In India, the ancient yogic tradition emphasizes that cooking fresh ingredients daily is not only tastier but also much healthier compared to buying packaged foods.

For dieting concerns, the main issue is often the feeling of constant hunger and the need to restrict certain foods. However, this is not true. Instead of depriving yourself, it's essential to rethink what you choose to nourish your body with.

A common excuse I often hear is that people don't want to go on a diet because they perceive it as too strict, and they fear it will deprive them of all the delicious food. They worry they will always feel hungry and unsatisfied. But is this true?

The key is to be smart about your choices. The best option is to cook your meals with fresh ingredients, as I mentioned before. My family and I do this daily because we enjoy it, not because we have free time or fear eating out.

I used to order takeout to save time, but after a week, it didn't taste as good as homemade food. Plus, if we didn't like it, what was the point? That's why my wife and I cook every day to have fresh meals on our table.

Now, let's explore different styles of dieting, as there are many options available for loss books. However, each style focuses on one specific aspect.

This overview was not intended to cover everything. Maybe you'll discover something new that suits you.

Let's inspect some popular diets like keto, Paleo, and intermittent fasting. Specifically, let's explore what the keto diet is all about a high-fat, adequate-protein, low-carbohydrate approach often used in medical settings to treat complex forms of epilepsy in children.

Beyond its medical origins, this diet essentially prompts the body to use fat as its primary energy source instead of carbohydrates. According to Wikipedia, the ketogenic diet involves consuming more calories from protein and fat and fewer carbohydrates. It focuses on incorporating more vegetables with meals rather than solely relying on meat and fat.

Similarly, people who follow the Paleo diet establish their eating habits on foods that they believe people consumed during the Paleolithic Era, such as meat, fish, vegetables, and fruit. In contrast, the Paleo diet excludes processed foods and cereal products. In short, these diets aim to mimic the eating habits of early humans, emphasizing a higher intake of protein and fat.

During the Paleolithic Era, our ancestors did not have access to processed foods like dairy products, cereals, and refined grains. As a result, their diet primarily comprised unprocessed vegetables, fruits, nuts, and meat. Many people who wish to avoid processed foods still follow this type of diet today. It typically includes vegetables, fruits, nuts, and meat while excluding dairy products, grains, legumes, processed oils, alcohol, and coffee. According to Wikipedia, people refer to this as a Paleo or cave dweller diet.

The major difference in this diet is that it focuses on eating individual foods rather than mixed dishes. For example, you would eat the meat separately from the vegetables instead of combining them in a dish.

This way of eating shares similarities with vegetarianism and veganism; both do not consume meat but may include eggs and dairy products in their diets. Vegetarians abstain from consuming meat, whereas vegans exclude not only meat but also any animal-derived products. This is the fundamental distinction between the two diets.

Let's discuss the Kettle diet, emphasizing low-carb choices and excluding grains like those in the Paleolithic diet. Similarly, widget adherents opt for mostly unprocessed foods, avoiding grains, legumes, and processed oils, resembling a cave dweller's diet in this sense. However, unlike their vegetarian counterparts, who may eat eggs or dairy occasionally, widget followers do not consume any animal products at all.

Now, there is a third option—the Mediterranean diet—which I tried and enjoyed. It features plenty of fresh produce and incorporates whole grains, legumes, healthy fats, and fish.

What does this entail? The general recommendation of this diet is to consume a diverse range of foods, including vegetables, fruits, and whole grains. It also incorporates four types of fats, such as nuts, seeds, and olive oil. In addition, the diet suggests a moderate intake of fish, limited consumption of white or red meat, occasional eggs, and some red wine.

People commonly practice the Mediterranean diet in Southern Europe because of its delicious and beneficial effects. This dietary approach includes consuming four types of fats, such as nuts, seeds, and olive oil. It suggests a moderate intake of fish, limited consumption of white or red meat, occasional eggs, and some red wine.

Another type of diet that has gained popularity is the low-carb diet, which restricts carbohydrates found in foods like bread. Instead, it focuses on high protein, fat, and nutrient-rich vegetables, such as lean meats (chicken breast or pork), fish, eggs, leafy greens (like cauliflower and broccoli), healthy fats (such as nut butter and oils), and some fruits (like apples, blueberries, and strawberries). To put it simply, no coarse bread, no pasta, or bars—but you can still enjoy these foods in moderation.

My favorite is intermittent fasting, which is not exactly a diet but an eating pattern with many benefits. So, what exactly are these diets? Have you heard of intermittent fasting?

It's a method where you alternate between periods of eating and not eating. The most popular approach is the 16:8 method, where you fast for 16 hours and then eat within an eight-hour window. Other common methods include the 5:2 diet, which involves alternating days of fasting and eating, or the 12-hour fast followed by a 12-hour eating period. While there are various types of intermittent fasting, the 16:8 method seems to be the most popular one.

I have tried this method myself, although now I do it for a slightly shorter amount of time each day. There are many benefits to intermittent fasting: it allows your body to repair itself and regulate gene expression, helps with weight loss and reduces visceral fat, can prevent type 2 diabetes, and promotes cardiovascular health by reducing insulin resistance and oxidative stress.

Besides potentially preventing cancer, incorporating intermittent fasting into your routine can help improve brain function and overall health. Experts recommend starting gradually, as your body may take some time to adjust to this type of fasting.

For example, beginning with a 14-hour fasting period from 6 p.m. to 8 a.m. the next morning may be more manageable than jumping straight into a longer fast.

I found that decreasing my fasting window by one hour each week was effective for me, eventually settling on a schedule of 17 hours fasting and 7 hours eating. This method has worked best for my body. Intermittent fasting also suits my lifestyle, since I don't require excessive amounts of food before going to the gym.

THINK OUT OF BELIEF

By not eating two hours before working out, I am less hungry during my workouts and have seen positive changes in my body composition thanks to intermittent fasting. I am very fond of this method. If you also enjoy it, conduct some research and give it a shot. It's not as challenging as it seems—simply gradually increases your fasting time, and you will find it quite doable to maintain consistently.

There is a general guideline for eating: ideally, your meals should comprise 1/3 carbohydrates (such as rice, potatoes, and bread), 1/3 protein, and 1/3 vegetables. I follow this rule almost every time I have lunch while practicing intermittent fasting.

However, explore and discover your unique approach. Experiment with these options and delve deeper into the subject by conducting further research. The results may pleasantly surprise you.

Numerous diets and lifestyles are options for selection. The key factor is using quality, natural, and possibly processed ingredients that are within your cooking abilities. You have the freedom to choose what you want to use. This method is the most effective in ensuring proper nutrition intake.

By being mindful of what you consume, researching, and selecting the best dietary option that interests you most—perhaps a video or one that is easily accessible—you can make informed choices. Make a list of necessary groceries, plan how to get them, and prepare accordingly. Take a chance and deliberately choose a dieting book that suits you well. Conduct further research by searching online or consulting with others to gather recipes for the specific style of dieting you wish to try.

Create a shopping list based on this and purchase the items. Give it a go! This will be your task until our next chapter: finding and gathering information while mentally preparing yourself for this change. What is necessary for you to believe and begin experiencing? I'll see you in our next lesson.

Summary: Takeaway Tips:

When we speak of dietary choices, we are not merely talking about food as fuel for the body. Food is life. How we consume and prepare it goes beyond health; it's about life. The ancients knew this well.

You see, food is not just a question of calories or nutrients. How we absorb the essence is significant. There are so many dietary styles out there: keto, Paleo, intermittent fasting—the list goes on.

Valid, but vital to grasp food must resonate with your body and mind. Our bodies are complex chemical systems, each of us a unique expression. What may work for one person may not work for another.

Therefore, I always say: don't believe what someone else tells you about food. Find out what works for you. The most important thing is to bring awareness to your food. The first step is to eliminate all processed foods.

Cook your meals. When you prepare your food, you infuse it with your energy. In yogic culture, they have always emphasized freshly cooking, preparing simple, and sattvic food that is rich in prana, the life force.

Explore different dietary styles, but understand that no matter what diet you choose, the fundamental rule is to eat consciously. When you eat consciously, you will know what is good for you.

Start with whole, unprocessed foods—vegetables, fruits, and grains—those that grow from the earth, nourished by the sun. Some of you might be interested in intermittent fasting.

Fasting is not just a diet; it's a way of giving your body the space to reset, repair, and rejuvenate. You are not simply depriving the body; you are allowing it to rest. When practiced mindfully, fasting becomes a powerful tool for health and well-being.

Remember, everybody is different. The food that nourishes you will differ from what nourishes another. The key is to explore, experiment, and listen to your body. Don't rush.

Approach it with reverence and see what truly works for you. Ultimately, the best diet is the one that brings harmony between your body, mind, and spirit. Food is not solely for energy. Make a wise choice and skip to chapter 8 for the three pillars of health.

Take a look at this table that illustrates the components of a scientifically proven balanced diet.

Nutrient Group	Key Components	Health Benefits
Carbohydrates	Whole grains (brown rice, oats, quinoa)	Provides energy, supports brain function, and promotes gut health.
	Fruits and vegetables (rich in fiber and vitamins)	
Proteins	Lean meats (chicken, turkey)	Builds and repairs tissues, supports muscle growth and immune function.
	Plant-based proteins (beans, lentils, tofu, chickpeas)	
Fats	Healthy fats (avocados, nuts, seeds, olive oil)	Supports brain health, hormone production, and cell structure.
	Omega-3 fatty acids (fish, flaxseeds, chia seeds)	Reduces inflammation, improves heart health.
Vitamins & Minerals	Vitamin-rich foods (leafy greens, citrus fruits, dairy products)	Boosts immunity, supports bone health, and improves skin and eye health.
	Mineral-rich foods (nuts, seeds, leafy vegetables)	
Fiber	Whole grains, fruits, vegetables, legumes	Promotes digestion, helps in weight management, and lowers cholesterol.
Water	Hydration through water, fruits, and	Maintains body temperature, flushes out toxins, and

vegetables   supports overall health.

Table 2

This table summarizes the components of a balanced diet and their benefits for maintaining overall health.

Chapter 8: The Three Pillars of Health and Well-Being: Emotion, Logic, and Physiology

****

"If you want something new, stop doing something old."–Peter F. Drucker

Have you heard of the three key components that make up health and well-being?

In Chapter 8, we will discuss the topic of whether to exercise. As a quick summary, we've already gone through the first two sections and are now moving on to the last two chapters. Do you recall our key point on how to lose weight easily? Keep in mind these three rules: know, decide, commit, be prepared for challenges.

We have already delved deeply into handling stress in previous chapters, so let's move on to another important aspect—nutrition. Remember to avoid gluten, lactose, and carbs for optimal health. Instead, focus on whole foods straight from the ground that haven't undergone processing. By following these simple guidelines, you will see the benefits for yourself.

The last chapter emphasizes three components for enhancing your overall health and well-being. These include the emotional, logical, and physiological aspects. Remember the triangle of hats? Let's start with the emotional component—finding meaning in your lifestyle choices.

Then there's the logical component, ensuring that we make educated decisions about our nutrition. And finally, there's the physiological component, also known as exercise or movement for our bodies. It's not just about losing weight or having a slim figure; it's about creating a lean and healthy body that you can feel good in.

Restricting your diet or doing stress-relieving exercises may cause weight loss, but it won't improve your body composition. I was once 213 pounds in one picture and 163 pounds in another, but neither reflected a healthy body composition that I was happy with.

Let's focus on creating a healthier and happier version of ourselves through three essential components. The experience revealed to me it wasn't as difficult as I thought.

Despite weighing 163 pounds, which may seem like a lot to some, many individuals are over 213 pounds and still feel confident and content. It wasn't the number on the scale that bothered me, but my body composition—the excess fat that I was carrying.

Even though losing just 4 pounds may not seem significant, compare the two photos with a difference of only 161 and 165 pounds, respectively; the change in body composition is clear. And this was all thanks to incorporating exercise into my routine.

If you want a lean, healthy body with lots of energy and to feel good in your skin, exercise should be part of your schedule. So instead of wondering if you should exercise or not, simply do it—for your health! Scientifically proven benefits include a reduced risk of diabetes, cancer, osteoarthritis, high blood pressure, and dementia, while also regulating existing conditions.

Health Condition	Benefit
Diabetes	Reduced risk of developing diabetes.
Cancer	Reduced risk of cancer.
Osteoarthritis	Reduced risk of osteoarthritis.
High Blood Pressure	Reduced risk of high blood pressure.
Dementia	Reduced risk of dementia.
Existing Conditions	Regulates and manages existing conditions (e.g., diabetes, blood pressure).

Table 3

Cardiovascular diseases are only one of the many health concerns that can arise if we neglect to take care of our bodies.

The list of potential risks is extensive, and it's important to be aware of how exercise can benefit us. Regular physical activity has a multitude of positive effects, both internally and externally. Not only will you feel better, but you'll also notice improvements in your appearance and self-confidence.

It's crucial to prioritize exercise for the sake of maintaining muscle mass; as the saying goes, "use it, or lose it." Building muscle gradually over time is key, rather than attempting extreme measures like training for a marathon right away.

However, this doesn't mean you have to push yourself beyond your limits immediately. Incorporating conscious exercise into your routine will make a significant difference in your overall well-being, just as being mindful of what you consume is important for your body's health. Let's make taking care of ourselves a conscious priority, both internally and externally.

Regular exercise can significantly improve your mood by triggering the release of happy hormones, such as dopamine and serotonin. The effectiveness is undeniable—observe those leaving our gym or engaging in gardening.

These happy hormones, including the powerful neurotransmitters dopamine and serotonin, play a crucial role in making us feel good. So, don't believe me outright; why not try exercise? Not only will it keep your mind sharp, but it will also increase your energy levels and enhance your social and sexual life. These benefits have been proven by researcher's time and again, and they are undeniably real.

However, with so many exercise books out there promising miraculous results, it's easy to get overwhelmed. Choose exercise based on personal preference. This aspect is vital because when we engage in activities we love, we are more likely to stick with them in the long run. So, start incorporating a physical activity into your routine today—your body and mind will thank you!

Cardio, strength, flexibility, balance, and coordination are all important components of exercise. There are endless options for different exercises, such as boxing, aerobics, yoga, Pilates, CrossFit, running, walking, football, swimming, hiking, stretching, mobility calisthenics, cycling, and more. Try a few to see which ones resonate most with you, my suggestion. You might find it surprising what you end up enjoying.

I remember when I first returned from China four and a half years ago and joined a nearby yoga class. If you want to include exercise in your routine like I did, why not give it a try? Initially, I wasn't using machines because I was out of shape and didn't feel comfortable jumping into other forms of exercise just yet.

However, now that I've found my rhythm, I realized that gardening alone wasn't cutting it for me, and I have been consistently exercising for quite some time now—it's safe to say that taking that initial step has certainly paid off in more ways than one!

During classes, everyone was jumping and using weights while upbeat music played in the background. I enjoyed the music but felt unprepared because of my lack of physical fitness. To address this, I incorporated a bit of walking, cycling, and other equipment-based exercises into my routine. However, these activities didn't appeal to me at all.

My wife suggested trying a combination class that included Tai Chi, and I found it to be much more enjoyable. For about a month, I mainly did yoga-inspired exercises but saw little change in my body, despite also improving my eating habits because of my inconsistency in practice. As my stomach continued to grow, I tried different classes. Group classes are better for me because of the instructor and other people.

Plus, it would have been too embarrassing for me to stand there alone while everyone else was taking part in the class. So now, I follow what everyone else is doing during these classes. I felt compelled to follow their tips, which motivated me to try new workouts. Through trial and error, I discovered that group exercise is my thing. I particularly enjoy combat-style classes, which I never would have expected at my age.

Discover an exercise that doesn't feel like work but brings joy and pride. Start slowly and gradually work your way up, whether that means joining a class or creating your workout routine on the gym floor.

Choose whatever form of exercise suits your best, whether it's running on the treadmill or focusing on your zone for relaxation or meditation purposes. Perhaps trying different exercise is the key. For me, group exercise classes have worked. No other reason could make me skip them; I enjoy them too much. It's not a chore, something I have to make myself do. Rather, it's something.

I look forward to, and my body is grateful for it. This was true in July, August, and November, when I could combine a variety of exercises. My advice to you is to explore different options because you never know what will fit your needs. Some prefer jumping on kangaroo-like structures, while others find joy in different creative workouts. Explore your surroundings and experiment until you discover what suits you.

Tried the gym, thought it'd be perfect, but wasn't my thing. However, this experience helped me narrow down the exercises I truly enjoy, and now I stick with them while adding in some strength training as well. For exercise, it's not just about doing strength training or just doing cardio.

Incorporating both types of exercise is beneficial for your body. Even if you are using your body weight, it can still have a positive impact on your body composition. I enjoy doing cardio exercises that I can do in the comfort of my home. It has helped my body transform quickly and effectively.

I suggest trying out different exercises to see what works best for you. Find the motivation to stick with the exercises that leave you feeling accomplished and mix it up with various classes as well.

This will help move your muscles in different ways and prevent boredom. Remember, exercise should be enjoyable, so do what make you happy and motivated to keep moving consistently. Whether it's gardening or simply taking a walk around the nearby locality, any form of movement is beneficial for your body. So just start somewhere and keep going–your body will thank you.

Summary: Take away tips

Ah, the three pillars of health and well-being – emotion, logic, and physiology. These paths are not separate, but rather three facets of one journey towards a balanced life.

When they are in harmony, you become capable of living fully, and health follows as a natural consequence. Every action you take is fueled by emotion.

How you feel, your moods and your aspirations all shape the choices you make each day. A lifestyle that nourishes your emotions will bring meaning and joy to every step of your journey.

Without emotion, life becomes a mechanical pursuit of goals. Therefore, allow yourself to feel deeply, engage passionately, and find meaning in the choices you make for your health.

Logic—the sharpness of the intellect—is your guide, your compass. It helps you discern what serves your well-being and what does not. In the realm of health, it is a logic that informs your decisions about nutrition, movement, and rest.

Logic shows you that consuming natural, whole foods, avoiding unnecessary indulgences, and practicing mindful eating are not restrictions but pathways to vitality.

Furthermore, there is physiology, which refers to the body itself. Your body is the temple in which this entire life experience unfolds. Through movement, it expresses itself; through stillness, it heals. Shaping the body through punishment is not the essence of exercise.

It's not just about appearance, but about being fully alive in every fiber of your being. When you bring these three elements—emotion, logic, and physiology—into balance, you create a life where health is not a goal but a natural expression of your existence.

Exercise, my friend, is not a question of "whether" but "how." How will you move your body today to align it with the joy and wisdom that lives within? Movement offers vast benefits for the body, mind, and spirit. It brings clarity, elevates your mood, and strengthens your connection to life. Take action with love, not burden. Let your exercise, your food, and your rest become sacred acts of self-care, and in doing so, you find that health, vitality, and joy naturally follow.

In Chapter 9, you will focus on the significance of rest, relaxation, and quality sleep in your weight loss journey.

Chapter 9: Rest, Rejuvenate, and Progress: The Power of Lazy Days and Quality Sleep.

******

"The real voyage of discovery consists not in thinking out of belief and seeking new landscapes, but in having fresh eyes."—*Marcel Proust.*

While this may initially aid in falling asleep, it can ultimately affect the quantity and quality of your rest. To truly rejuvenate, it is best to sleep in a dark and quiet room, giving your brain and body the relaxation. So be sure to choose a peaceful setting for your sleep rather than compromising with distractions.

Ensuring quality sleep is crucial for rejuvenating your muscles and being your major source of energy. To have a relaxed and healthy body, it's important to prioritize lazy days and getting enough sleep. Listen to your body's internal clock and aim for sufficient rest. However, this doesn't mean staying until 3 a.m. every night. Your body is intelligent and adapts to its surroundings, but this is not how we function. Our natural rhythm involves a balance of rest and activity.

It may be beneficial to experiment with going to bed earlier, perhaps at 11 p.m., and observe the effects on your energy levels, mood, and mental clarity the following day. Bedtime before midnight can significantly affect your overall physical and mental state. Relax and take things slowly.

Keep in mind, it's not a competition, but a marathon. Each step is important as you embark on this journey of self-improvement. Don't worry; it's simple and manageable. You're just beginning to understand and implement this process in your life. So, keep calm and persevere toward success. Enjoy the journey without stressing over the end result. Take a deep breath, relax, and remember—easy, do it.

No rush doesn't overwhelm yourself with everything. Start by trying fresh foods, diets, stress-relief techniques such as meditation or tapping points, and activities like walking or gardening.

If that's what you want, don't worry about it seeming like a lot initially—just do it. You shouldn't let anyone stop you from watching some mindless TV but try not to get too invested in it. I also sometimes indulge in watching soap operas or reading both good and bad books that offer an escape from daily life. However, it's important not to get too caught up in all of it.

Start slowly and take it easy as you make changes. Don't feel you need to rush or hurry; just focus on your journey one step at a time. It's not realistic to expect immediate results within a week or even a month, as our current state reflects years of habits and possibly emotional stress.

Change takes time, and that's okay. Allow yourself time to understand and implement this book without feeling overwhelmed. Remember, progress takes time, but as long as you keep you will eventually reach your goal. So don't worry or stress about it; just relax and start taking small steps toward your success.

In addition, I have two pieces of advice for you. The first and most crucial one is to focus on your path. Avoid comparing yourself to others or feeling impatient with the progress of those around you. I have made this mistake myself, fixating on someone else's body and feeling discouraged about my progress. But it's important to remember that we all have different starting points and ways of reaching our goals. You never know what sacrifices or resources others may use to achieve their results.

What truly matters is focusing on your own growth and progress, without comparing yourself to anyone else.

What matters most is that you don't compare yourself to anyone else, and don't be too hard on yourself if you fall behind your plan. Drifting from a set plan can be beneficial because it helps identify the steps needed to reach your desired outcome, although plans can also cause stress if used as a measuring stick against others. Remember to stay focused on your journey and trust your unique process toward success.

Oh, my goodness, I should be at 163 pounds by now, but I'm currently at 167 pounds. So, what am I doing wrong? Well, nothing at all. It's important to remember that changes in our bodies take time. Perhaps it's taking longer than you expected, or there may still be some missing pieces or factors that need to align. Your body simply needs more time to recognize and adapt to the changes you desire.

Don't let comparisons bring you down, it's just part of life. Everyone's journey is unique, and that doesn't make yours any less valid. The key is to concentrate on your progress and proceed at your own pace and style.

Slow and steady wins the race, so don't rush or get discouraged if change doesn't happen overnight. Ultimately, setting a goal and sticking to it is what truly matters, not comparing yourself to others or being impatient with the process. Create a plan to achieve your goals at your own pace while managing stress and minding your own business. There's no need for others to be aware or rush yourself. Take control of the situation, and you will undoubtedly find success.

Remember, it's perfectly acceptable to have days when you simply relax—whether that means doing nothing but sitting on the sofa with a good or bad book or indulging in mindless television shows. We all need a break from our daily routines, and television can serve as a helpful tool for that purpose. The key is to prioritize relaxation and ensure you get enough quality sleep. Aim for bedtime between 10 P.M. and 6 A.M., and make sure your room is comfortably dark and cool. When working towards weight loss, it's crucial to focus on your progress without getting distracted by external factors or comparing yourself to others.

Your body is constantly changing, and that, in itself, is a success. Remember, change takes time. Patience is key for your body's transformation. Instead of stressing overachieving your goal quickly, appreciate the journey and value yourself along the way. Take lazy days as an opportunity to relax and rejuvenate both mentally and physically, allowing your muscles to become stronger. So, enjoy these days guilt-free; you deserve them.

The Transformation Blueprint is a holistic approach that provides a clear framework for transforming one's life and achieving desired goals. My Journey to a Healthier Life.

In this chapter 10, I share my journey of transformation, highlighting the steps I took to achieve a healthier body and mindset. The chapter emphasizes the importance of visualizing success, making dietary changes, managing carbohydrate intake, incorporating intermittent fasting, and dealing with stress in healthy ways.

It also discusses the significance of finding joy in fitness, staying motivated, and celebrating the progress made on the path to a healthier lifestyle. Welcome back to your final chapter, number 10. As previously promised, I will reveal the specific steps I took to transform my body from where it was to where it is now.

This process only took a few months for me and is still ongoing. Now, let me show how I achieved the most effective change in body composition. My approach may not be the same as yours, as you are free to choose your own path toward reaching your desired weight and body composition. Let me take you through the steps once again, as I am currently making changes myself. I understand that this may seem repetitive but trust me when I say it's important information that deserves to repeat.

Recall the simple approach to losing weight. By adhering to three rules, you must understand the steps and put them into practice, beginning with adjusting your diet. Take charge of your mindset and cope with stress. Next, make better food choices in place of unhealthy ones, and engage in physical activity, as evidenced by the triangle of wellness at play. It all boils down to managing your emotions, making wiser nutritional decisions, and incorporating movement and rest into your daily routine.

Allow me to show my success using this method. Change the Appearance. This remains one of my favorite photos, and as previously suggested, I highly recommend keeping both your best and most unflattering shots. I'm thankful that I still have this photo because it serves as a great visual aid for tracking my progress. Initially, I deleted it because of its poor quality, but then recovered it. Printing it out will serve as a tangible reminder of my journey.

Seeing that photo helps me stay motivated and determined to never revert to my previous state. It was a clear sign I needed to make some changes in my lifestyle. Yes, I wasn't 213 pounds, but for myself and my friend, it was incredibly embarrassing. After seeing a photo of myself on holiday in July, I had finally reached my breaking point. I was tired of my current appearance and knew I needed to make a permanent change back to my normal self.

I understand if you want to bring up my previous struggles with obesity, but that shouldn't stop us from striving for a better version of ourselves. We can't use our busy lifestyles as an excuse because we need the energy to keep up with them. That's why.

I made the final decision to take full control of my body. That picture was the breaking point for me. Excuses were no longer an option for me. After returning from China, I was determined to improve my body to the best of my ability. One change I made was cutting out carbohydrate-rich foods, gluten, and lactose.

While I do not have any symptoms related to these foods, my family and I decided it was important for our overall health. Therefore, I strictly avoided carbohydrate-rich foods, gluten, and lactose to maintain a healthy lifestyle for all of us. This included cleaning up my diet, reducing my carbohydrate intake to a minimum, and saying no to gluten and lactose, without exception.

Do I still eat foods that are rich in carbohydrates? Without a doubt.

However, the amount I consume now is negligible compared to how much I used to eat. Chocolate is still a part of my diet because I am a man and I enjoy it, but I prefer dark chocolate with at least 85% cocoa. Some days, a small piece is enough, while other days, it may not be. Occasionally, I will have some raisins for a touch of sweetness.

Being a man, I appreciate the taste of carb treats, but my intake has significantly decreased from what it used to be. This is something that continues even during the holidays. Interestingly enough, for the past four and a half years, I have had the same breakfast every day, and yet, I am not tired of it.

It leaves me satisfied and deliciously fulfilled, and it's beneficial for my health as well. I have enough energy to last me until lunchtime. For breakfast, I stick to the same routine, and if you're interested, I'll share the recipe in the previous section. It was a firm decision of mine to cut out carbs and focus on protein instead, which has become a regular meal for us—either for dinner or lunch. And let me tell you, it's delicious and satisfying.

Another change I made was incorporating intermittent fasting into my routine. I fast for 10 to 12 hours each day and became strict with my eating schedule. Initially, I only ate between 8 PM and 8 AM. I must confess, I occasionally have cheat days when I eat a bit later, but never past 8:00 PM. This means that there are some mornings when I don't eat until 7:54 AM, as my body has become accustomed to intermittent fasting. Going to bed early also helps curb any hunger pangs.

I have handled stress, such as playing with my beloved dog or son and using ESR whenever and wherever necessary. We often head to the forest valley side for exercise and fun activities. In this way, I can healthily manage stress and enjoy quality time with my loved ones.

Initially, I struggled with ESR and self-sabotage, as well as tapping and goal setting while planning and focusing on my overall well-being. However, the speed at which I achieved my desired results was not a major concern for me, considering I already had a job.

Therefore, the pressures of children and deadlines did not dictate my progress. Instead, I made a personal decision to change for myself, regardless of how long it took.

Fortunately, within the first five years, I noticed a significant change in both my physical and mental state. Although it took me almost a year to reach my desired body composition, it was worth the journey, as I now feel more comfortable in my skin.

Through consistency and dedication to regular gym sessions and taking part in group exercise classes that promote camaraderie with like-minded individuals, led by knowledgeable instructors, I found joy in following structured programs tailored to my liking. The music is excellent, and I've grown to love the experience of combining combat, yoga, and core training.

Initially, I had reservations about yoga being too slow and combat and jogging being too intense but incorporating them all has surprisingly resulted in a satisfying workout. With these classes, I never have to force myself to go, except for a few occasions during winter when it's dark and cold outside.

On those days, I push through because once I'm there; I feel proud and accomplished. That's why I've been a member of this yoga club for four years now—the classes are simply wonderful.

Initially, I was overweight and didn't feel good about it. I made excuses for myself, like lack of energy, time, and motivation. But after a while, I realized that enough was enough and made a change. And guess what? It has made all the difference. Now my body has gone from being small to smaller because I am also making healthy changes.

And the best part is that I have continued this journey and am still going strong. I don't walk every day, but it has become a regular part

Summary: Takeaway Tips:

In this journey of transformation, we do not separate the body and mind.

The steps you take are not just physical actions—they are profound shifts in the way you experience life.

Visualizing success is not mere imagination; it is planting the seed of what you wish to become.

The food you eat, the rest you take, and the stillness you find—these are not simply habits, but the architecture of a balanced life.

In my journey, I learned that reducing carbs, fasting, and managing stress were not just methods; they were ways to reclaim harmony within myself.

Fitness became not a task, but a joyful expression of life's vitality.

As you walk your path, remember this: health is not a destination—it is a way of being, one that is always developing.

We can shape the body, sculpt the mind, and find joy even in the smallest of steps.

Let your transformation be a dance of discipline and grace, and celebrate every moment of progress, for that is where genuine change lives.

This is your journey, your blueprint—embrace it with both humility and courage.

Explore my upcoming books that delve into the diverse spectrum of personal experiences in different life stages.

Stay connected and let stories that resonate with every stage of life inspire you. Join me on this journey and enrich your own!

Thank you.

Chapter-NXR: Be among the first to read the gripping first chapter of my eagerly awaited new book

Challenge yourself to think outside the boundaries of old age." Introductory story.

The Last Sunset:

The sun was setting on another quiet evening when Mikel, a frail 75-year-old, sat slumped in his armchair by the window, watching the fading light. Years of sorrow had etched deep lines on his face—hardship and the cruelties of life had carved them, taking more from him than he ever thought possible.

Once a vibrant man, Mikel had become a shadow of himself, his spirit dimmed by betrayal and loneliness. His life savings, looted by a Thai woman he had trusted, left him not only penniless but broken in ways that money could never mend.

The old-age home where Mikel now lived was a place of routine, where days and nights blurred together in a monotony that stripped away the dignity of older adults. It was a sterile waiting room for death, a place where people like Mikel faded, forgotten by the world. They denied his appeal for assisted death, leaving him with nothing but three days to endure before he could carry out his final plan on his terms.

Mikel's home, once filled with his children's laughter, was now too painful to return to. His wife's warmth had long since vanished from his life, leaving behind only cold, haunting memories. His heart could no longer bear the weight of those ghosts, and he knew he could never step foot in that house again.

He wanted freedom—not the kind found in the flickering light of a television screen or the mundane pleasantries of well-meaning caregivers—but the freedom to feel alive once more. To be in a place where the air carried the scent of flowers, and they sunbathed him in warmth. But as night fell, Mikel knew that such a place, such peace, seemed beyond his reach.

In those last few days, as he held the prescription pills in his hand, he did not truly think out of belief and seek death but escape—from the system that had reduced his life to a routine of pills and paperwork, and from a body that had become a prison.

The system, cold and indifferent, seemed to strip away not just the dignity of older adults but the essence of life itself. Mikel's desire to die was not the despair of someone afraid of life; it was the deep yearning of a man who had lost everything and had nothing left to fight for.

He no longer believed in the system. He wanted to walk free, feel the earth under his feet, and breathe the air of a place where he could truly live again.

So, on the third day of his silent commitment, after the pills offered no solace, he journeyed to India—a land he had only heard about, a place of believers, seekers, and healers, where life could be discovered not by avoiding pain but by transcending it. He sought the embrace of a community where healing came not from medicine but from a deeper connection to life itself. It was as though his soul knew, long before his mind did, that his last journey was not to death but to life itself—where life and death are two sides of the same coin.

In the land of think out of believer but seekers, where spiritual traditions run deep, Mikel found his way to an ashram nestled in the foothills of the mountains.

He stepped into a space where the material world no longer held him, where the sun and wind were his companions, and where each breath was a reminder of the vitality he had long forgotten.

When he arrived at the gates, frail and exhausted, a young sadhu greeted him with folded hands and a warm smile. "Welcome, stranger," the sadhu said. "This is a place of healing. You have come to the right place."

The ashram, with its serene gardens and soft chants echoing through the trees, enveloped Mikel in a peace he hadn't known for reviews and certain other non-commercial uses permitted by copyright law.

Disclaimer

The author intends for the information provided in this book to be for general knowledge and educational purposes only. It is not a substitute for professional medical advice, diagnosis, or treatment. The author is not a licensed healthcare provider, and the content of this book should not be medical advice.

Before changing your diet, exercise routine, or health practices based on the recommendations in this book, please consult with a qualified healthcare professional. Every individual's health needs and conditions are unique, and what works for one person may not be suitable for another.

The author and publisher are not liable for any damages, injuries, or health-related issues that may arise from following the suggestions or strategies outlined in this book. By reading and applying the information in this book, you assume full responsibility for any outcomes or consequences that may result.

References:

1.Sadh **guru** (**Jaggi Vasudev**). *Inner Engineering: A Yogi's Guide to Joy*. New York: Spiegel & Grau, 2016.

2. Sadh **guru** (**Jaggi Vasudev**). *Karma: A Yogi's Guide to Crafting Your Destiny*. New York: Harmony Books, 2021.

3.Chip **Heath** and **Dan Heath**. *Decisive: How to Make Better Choices in Life and Work*. New York: Crown Business, 2013.

4.Charles **Duhigg**. *The Power of Habit: Why We Do What We Do in Life and Business*. New York: Random House, 2012.

5.Eckhart Tolle. *The Power of Now: A Guide to Spiritual Enlightenment*. Novato, CA: New World Library, 1997.

6.Deepak Chopra. *Perfect Health: The Complete Mind Body Guide*. New York: Three Rivers Press, 1991.

7.Don Miguel Ruiz. *The Four Agreements: A Practical Guide to Personal Freedom*. San Rafael, CA: Amber-Allen Publishing, 1997.

9 798227 451309